Table of Contents

INTRODUCTION

Inflammation and infection of diverticula are called diverticulitis. Diverticula are pouches which occur along the digestive tract, most often in the colon (large intestine). These pouches are formed when weak spots in the intestine balloon outward. The process of forming pouches is called diverticulosis. Diverticulitis is a more serious condition when these pouches get infected by bacteria and eventually get inflamed causing perforation of the bowel. The pouches commonly form at the end of the descending and sigmoid colons located on the left side of the abdomen. They also mostly occur in the first section of the small intestine, which rarely causes problems. Diverticula are generally harmless. People having diverticula which are not infected is called diverticulosis.

Diverticulosis typically causes no symptoms and does not need treatment. Only 10-20% of people having diverticulosis progress to a condition called symptomatic uncomplicated diverticular disease (SUDD) and the symptoms are similar to irritable bowel syndrome, which includes abdominal pain and bloating. Typically it takes about 7 years for symptomatic uncomplicated diverticular disease (SUDD) to progress to diverticulitis.

Disease progression

An episode of diverticulitis can usually recur as an acute, or short-term, problem. However, there is no definite timeframe. Studies have shown that when a person has an episode of diverticulitis, he or she is more likely to have another episode of an acute attack within five years. Usually, the first attack is the worst one because scar tissue builds up in the diverticula and helps prevent future perforations. If the first episode is mild, there is a higher chance of avoiding serious complications. There are also cases when diverticulitis can progress into a chronic or long-term problem. These cases can be much more serious and surgery may be required to remove the diseased tissue.

Risk factors

There are several risk factors associated with diverticulitis. The foremost risk factor can be associated with age. There is a higher risk of developing diverticulitis at an older age. Diverticulosis, which is the predecessor to diverticulitis, is quite common in adults, especially people above the age of 60. Studies have estimated that diverticulitis can affect 60% of people over age 70 and can affect 75% of people who are 80 years and older. People who are diagnosed very early with diverticulosis have a higher chance of progression to diverticulitis later in their life.

Causes of diverticulitis

One of the main causes of diverticulitis is by fecal matter blocking the opening of diverticula. This can cause inflammation and infection. It can vary from person to person. Multiple factors can lead to diverticulitis, which is discussed below:

- Low-fiber diet: People consuming a low fiber diet are at higher risk of developing diverticulitis. Studies have shown that a lack of dietary fiber has long been suspected for the onset of diverticulitis.

- Heredity: Heredity seems to play an important part for people to have diverticulitis. Research has shown that more than 50% of the potential risk of diverticular disease comes from genetics.

- Obesity: Obesity is another factor related to diverticulitis. People who are obese have a clear risk factor for diverticulitis. Obesity raises the risk of diverticulitis and bleeding, but there is no clear reason behind this.

- Lack of Physical Exercise: People having a sedentary lifestyle are more prone to diverticulitis. Exercise helps a person be flexible and helps in muscle contraction and extension, which is required for a healthy intestine. A sedentary lifestyle can hamper this process, which can lead to the onset of disease.

- Smoking: Research has shown that smoking can increase the risk of symptomatic and complicated diverticular disease.

- Medications People who consume prescribed medications such as aspirin and other nonsteroidal anti-inflammatory drugs (NSAIDs) have a higher risk of diverticulitis. The use of opiates and steroids raises the risk of perforation, which is a serious complication of diverticulitis.

- Vitamin D deficiency: Studies have also noted that people with complicated diverticulitis tend to have lower levels of vitamin D. Studies suggest that vitamin D levels seem to be related to complications of the disease.

- Age and Sex: Diverticulitis seems to be more common among people with the age group of 50 and younger. Diverticulitis also appears to be slightly more common in men than women in this age group. Diverticulitis seems more common in women who are older than 50 years.

Symptoms of Diverticulosis and Diverticulitis

People having diverticulosis usually have minimal to no symptoms. Diverticula are generally painless and hardly cause any symptoms. Some of the symptoms of diverticulosis are:

- Cramping on the left side of the abdomen. This disappears after passing gas or moving the bowels.
- Bright red blood in the stool.

Diverticulitis symptoms are much noticeable. Pain in the abdomen is the most common symptom, which typically occurs in the lower left side of the abdomen. Diverticulitis most often affects the part of the colon in that area. The most common symptoms of diverticulitis include fever, nausea, abdominal pain, vomiting, burning sensation while urinating, increased urge to urinate, constipation, and diarrhea.

Blood in the stool, as well as bleeding from the rectum, occurs in both diverticulosis and diverticulitis. Diverticulitis may be acute or chronic. The acute form of diverticulitis can display itself with one or more severe attacks of infection and inflammation. The infection may never clear up completely in the case of chronic diverticulitis but may subside. The inflammation that is caused can eventually result in a bowel obstruction, which may cause abdominal swelling or bloating, constipation, thin stools, diarrhea, and abdominal pain. When obstruction persists, abdominal pain and tenderness will increase and people may experience nausea and vomiting.

Complications of Diverticulitis

Diverticulitis can lead to serious complications if untreated and may even require surgery. Some of the complications associated with diverticulitis include:

- Abscesses may form around the infected diverticula. These abscesses go through the intestinal wall and people may develop peritonitis, which is potentially a fatal infection, which requires immediate treatment.

- Scarring may occur, leading to a stricture or blockage of the intestine.
- Fistulas are formed when an infected diverticulum reaches an adjoining organ. This generally occurs between the large intestine and the bladder.
- May require transfusion if the bleeding is severe.

Treatment for diverticulitis

Diverticulitis is usually a medical emergency depending on the severity of symptoms and may require immediate medical attention and admission to the hospital whereas mild attacks can be treated at home.

- No eating or drinking. Intravenous fluids are given for the bowel to rest.
- Pain-relieving medication.
- Surgery may be needed in severe cases when the weakened sections of the bowel wall have

ruptured or become obstructed, or if the attack of infection fails to settle.

- Doctors try to rejoin the healthy section of the bowel during surgery and if it is not possible to rejoin the healthy sections of bowel, a colostomy bag will be fitted. This is generally temporary and the bowel can be rejoined after six to 12 months.

- Long-term use of mild antibiotic becomes necessary to prevent further attacks.

Foods to avoid

1. High-FODMAP foods: FODMAP foods are called as fermentable oligosaccharides, disaccharides, monosaccharides, and polyols food. Research has shown that a diet, which limits foods that are high in FODMAP, can benefit people with irritable bowel syndrome, which is one of the common symptoms of diverticulitis. Foods high in FODMAPs include:

   o Fruits, such as apples, pears, and plums.

- Dairy foods, such as yogurt, ice cream, and milk.
    - Fermented foods, such as sauerkraut or kimchi.
    - Brussels sprouts.
    - Onions and garlic.
2. High-fiber foods: Foods that are high in fiber usually are very helpful for people with diverticulosis as well as diverticulitis. A systematic review showed a reduction of abdominal symptoms and the prevention of acute diverticulitis with the intake of fiber diet.

However, different people react in different ways depending on the symptoms they have due to the specific fiber needs, which varies based on the condition and symptoms. Doctors generally ask people to avoid these high fiber foods if the person is having pain or other symptoms.

Fiber adds bulk to stool and may increase peristalsis or colon contractions, which may be painful and uncomfortable when having a flare-up. Avoiding high-fiber foods in such cases may ease symptoms and give the system a temporary rest.

Fiber-rich foods which need to be avoided during a flare-up include:

- Beans and legumes such as kidney beans, chickpeas, navy beans, lentils.
- Whole grains such as quinoa, oats, brown rice, etc.

3. Foods High in Sugar and Fat: Diet containing a high amount of sugar and fat are generally not advisable for any medical condition. A diet containing high in fat and sugar and low in fiber may be linked with an increased incidence of diverticulitis. Some of the foods, which can be avoided to prevent diverticulitis include:
   - Red meat.
   - Refined grains.
   - Full-fat dairy.
   - Fried foods.

4. Other foods to avoid: Doctors generally advise not to consume foods such as nuts, popcorn, and most seeds. Since tiny particles from these

foods might get lodged in the pouches and lead to an infection, they are generally avoided. There is no stern evidence that these foods may lead to diverticulitis, but just an assumption. Research has also suggested that people with diverticulitis should avoid alcohol.

Foods to eat

There are some foods, which the doctor recommends to manage diverticulitis. Treatment and disease management for diverticulitis vary from person to person. Change in diet may help people to have lesser symptoms and limit recurrence. During an acute attack of diverticulitis, the doctor may suggest either a low-fiber diet or a clear liquid diet to help relieve the symptoms.

1. Low-fiber foods to consider during the symptoms of diverticulitis include:
   - White rice, white bread, or white pasta, but avoid gluten-containing foods if you're intolerant

- Dry, low-fiber cereals

- Processed fruits

- Cooked animal proteins

- Olive oil or other oils

- Yellow squash, zucchini, or pumpkin: peeled, seeds removed, and cooked

- Cooked spinach, beets, carrots, or asparagus

- Potatoes with no skin.

- Fruit and vegetable juices.

2. Clear liquid diet: A clear liquid diet is the first choice of diet administered during hospitalization to relieve diverticulitis symptoms. A clear liquid diet is prescribed for a short period of time and may consist:

- Ice chips.

- Ice pops with frozen fruit puree or pieces of finely chopped fruit.

- Soup broth or stock.

- Gelatin, such as Jell-O.

- Tea or coffee excluding any creams, flavors, or sweeteners.

- Clear electrolyte drinks.

- Drinking at least eight cups of water daily seems to be the ideal choice when following any diet. Drinking adequate amount of water helps you keep hydrated and supports gastrointestinal health. Usually, after a prescription of clear liquid diet for a few days, doctors may recommend slowly adding low-fiber foods back into the diet.

Once the symptoms of diverticulitis have subsided, doctors may suggest resuming a balanced diet.

Some Simple Steps to Help Prevent Diverticulitis

Other than diet, there are several other ways you can maintain good digestive health and prevent diverticula from forming, including avoiding eating too much red meat, avoiding fatty foods, and drinking plenty of fluids.

Nonsteroidal anti-inflammatory drugs (NSAIDs), such as aspirin, Aleve (naproxen), and Advil or Motrin (ibuprofen) have been linked to increased instances of diverticular bleeding.

High-fiber diets need water to function properly. If you don't drink enough water, you can put yourself at greater risk of constipation.

Finally, delaying bowel movements can lead to hard stools and increased strain on the muscles of the colon, which may lead to diverticular disease.

Here are some habits to practice to avoid diverticulitis:

- Exercise regularly
- Quit smoking (smokers are at a higher risk of developing complications from diverticulitis)
- Avoid the use of NSAIDs
- Drink plenty of fluids
- Maintain a healthy body weight
- Respond to bowel urges
- Moderate red meat intake

Sample Meal Plan

Breakfast

- fruit juice
- wholemeal bread or toast with boiled egg, or spread (butter, jam without pips etc)

Lunch

- tuna sandwich with wholemeal bread
- plain or flavoured yoghurt (avoid fruit yoghurts with pips)
- piece of fruit

Dinner

- vegetable soup
- chicken with steamed potatoes (without the skin) and vegetables.
- fruit

RECIPES

Low FODMAP French Oven Beef Stew

Often times, diets can feel restrictive and exhausting. This beef stew recipe is far from boring and will surely satisfy you. Some vegetables are high FODMAP foods such as garlic, asparagus, cauliflower and several others that can make eating a wholesome meal feel confusing and possibly difficult. Rest assured, this recipe contains low FODMAP veggies, is hearty and is a perfect comfort food meal. This hearty and nourishing Low FODMAP French Oven Beef Stew is a great way to eat a variety of vegetables in one meal. Perfect for winter!

Prep Time: 15 minutes

Cook Time: 4 hours

Servings: 6

Ingredients

- 1 lb beef for stew
- 1 cup fennel bulb , diced
- 1 medium celery stalks

- 6 medium carrots
- 4 medium parsnips
- 4 medium potatoes
- 1/4 cup tapioca quick cooking
- 1 cup tomato juice
- 1 Tbsp sugar (optional)
- ½ tsp salt
- ½ tsp freshly ground pepper
- 1 tsp ground basil

Instructions

1. Preheat oven to 300°F. Cut the beef into approximately 4 cm/1 ½ inch cubes.
2. Wash all vegetables well. Scrub potato skin to remove all dirt. Medium dice celery stalks and fennel bulb. Chop carrots, parsnips and potatoes into medium sized pieces.
3. Mix all ingredients EXCEPT potatoes in a large oven-safe dish with a lid. Cover and bake in oven for 3 hours.
4. Mix in potatoes and bake for 1 hour longer. Enjoy!

Notes

- Make sure to purchase tomato juice WITHOUT added onion or garlic
- If your tomato juice is sodium-free, option to increase amount of salt to 1 tsp
- Fennel bulb is low FODMAP at 1/2 cup per serving. Celery is low FODMAP at 1/4 medium stalk per serving. There is 1 medium celery stalk in the stew and therefore the max FODMAP serving size is 1/4 of the recipe; this means that you could eat up to 1/4 of the total amount of stew and still stay low FODMAP.

Blueberry Breakfast Bars

Prep Time: 5 minutes

Cook Time: 25 minutes

Total Time: 30 minutes

Yield: 9 squares

Serving Size: 1 sqaure

Ingredients

Bottom layer:

- 2 cups large flake oats
- 4 tbsp pure maple syrup
- 2 ripe bananas
- 1 scoop (1/4 cup) FODMAP friendly protein powder (such as BOOST Just Protein whey protein isolate)
- 1 tsp cinnamon powder
- 2 tsp coconut oil
- 1/4 tsp salt

Top layer:

- 1 cup blueberries
- 1/2 cup large flake oats
- 1/3 cup pumpkin seeds
- 1/4 cup chopped walnuts
- 2 tbsp chia seeds
- 1/2 tsp cinnamon powder
- 1/4 cup almond milk

Instructions

1. Preheat an oven to 350°F. Line a 9 x 9 inch baking dish with parchment paper and spray lightly with cooking spray.
2. In a food processor, combine all ingredients of bottom layer. Pulse until smooth and wet; about 1 minute. Transfer into the lined baking dish, and spread evenly and firmly into all four corners with a spatula. Place in preheated oven and bake for 10 minutes.
3. In a medium bowl, combine remaining top layer ingredients; mix well.
4. Remove baking pan from oven, and top with blueberry mixture. Push berry mixture into all corners of pan and press down firmly. Place back in oven for 15 minutes.
5. Remove and let cool, then cut into 9 squares.

Sheet Pan Fajitas

Prep Time: 10 mins

Cook Time: 30 mins

Total Time: 40 mins

Yield: 4 servings

Ingredients

- 1 sweet potato, cleaned and chopped into quarter size pieces
- 2 bell peppers, sliced into strips
- 2 zucchinis, sliced into strips
- 3 carrots, sliced into strips
- 2 chicken breasts, cut into bite-sized pieces
- 2 Tbsp smoked paprika
- 1 Tbsp dried chives
- 1 1/2 tsp salt
- 1 1/2 tsp ground cumin
- 1 tsp dried oregano
- 1/4 tsp black pepper
- 1 Tbsp extra virgin olive oil

Instructions

1. Preheat oven to 400 degrees fahrenheit.
2. Combine all ingredients in a large bowl or zip-top bag (you may need to do this in two bowls or bags depending on size).
3. Spread the seasoned vegetables and chicken on 1-2 sheet pans (again depending on size) so that it is laying in an even layer without too much crowding or overlap.
4. Roast at 400 degrees for 30 minutes (stirring at the 15 minute mark) or until the chicken is cooked to 165 degrees fahrenheit.
5. Serve as is, with whole grain tortillas, tortilla chips, or however you like.

Notes

This is a great meal for meal prep! Simply chop all the veggies and chicken ahead of time and you are more than halfway to dinner time!

Nutrition

- Serving Size: 1/4 recipe
- Calories: 261
- Sugar: 6 g
- Sodium: 787 mg
- Fat: 7 g
- Carbohydrates: 15 g
- Protein: 33 g

Banana Nut Oatmeal Muffins

Prep Time: 20 minutes

Cook Time: 35 minutes

Total Time: 55 minutes

Servings 12 muffins

Ingredients

- 2 large ripe bananas
- 2 1/2 cups quick oats (gluten-free if needed)
- 1 1/2 cups lactose-free milk (almond milk for dairy-free)

- 1/4 cup pure maple syrup
- 1 large egg, lightly beaten
- 2 tablespoons canola oil
- 1 teaspoon baking powder
- 1 1/2 teaspoons ground cinnamon
- 1 teaspoon vanilla extract
- 1/4 teaspoon salt
- 1/2 cup chopped walnuts
- 1/4 cup Enjoy Life Dairy-Free Mini Chocolate Chips (or finely chopped dark chocolate)

Instructions

1. Heat oven to 350 degrees F and coat a 12-count non-stick muffin tin with cooking spray.
2. In a large bowl, mash the bananas with a fork. Add the oats and milk. Stir until evenly combined. Let soak about 5 to 10 minutes, or until most of the liquid is absorbed.
3. To the oat mixture, add the maple syrup, egg, canola oil, baking powder, cinnamon, vanilla and salt. Stir until thoroughly combined. Stir in the walnuts and chocolate or chocolate chips.

4. Fill each muffin cup with approximately 1/3 cup of the batter. Bake for 30 to 35 minutes or until lightly browned and tops spring back when lightly touched in the middle on top. Cool in pan for 10 minutes, then remove to cooling rack.

5. Refrigerate leftover muffins for up to 2 days or freeze for up to 3 months in an airtight, resealable bag.

Mediterranean Grilled Cheese

Prep Time: 5 minutes

Cook Time: 10 minutes

Total Time: 15 minutes

Yield: 1

Ingredients

- 2 teaspoons butter

- 2 slices low FODMAP bread, such as Schär Deli Style Seeded Bread
- 2 Roma tomato slices
- ¼ cup spinach leaves
- 2 tablespoons pitted Kalamata olives
- 1 ounce (28 grams) sliced fresh mozzarella
- 1 tablespoon (10 grams) feta cheese

INSTRUCTIONS

1. Spread butter evenly onto both sides of each piece of low FODMAP bread.
2. To one slice of bread, add the tomato slices, spinach, olives, mozzarella, and feta. Finish with the second slice of bread.
3. Preheat sandwich press (or skillet over medium heat). Once hot, grill the sandwich (or cook in the skillet, flipping after 2-3 minutes per side) until bread is golden brown and cheese is melted.
4. Serve warm.

Chocolate Chip Cookies

These cookies are soft and gooey, but still lightly browned on the bottom and firm enough to dunk in milk or tea. Truly the best chocolate chip cookies!

Servings 36 cookies

Ingredients

- 1/2 cup butter softened
- 1/2 cup sugar
- 1/2 cup packed brown sugar
- 1 large egg
- 1/4 teaspoon salt
- 1 teaspoon vanilla
- 1/2 cup white rice flour
- 3 tbsp sweet/glutinous rice flour
- 3 tbsp tapioca starch
- 1/2 tsp xantham gum
- 1/4 cup almond flour
- 1/2 teaspoon baking soda
- 3/4 cup chocolate chips

Instructions

1. Preheat the oven to 325°F. Cover a baking sheet with parchment paper.

2. Place butter in a bowl at room temperature for 30 minutes. Alternative: heat butter in the microwave on low until just softened but not melted.

3. Cream the butter and sugars together in a large bowl using a fork until well combined. Beat in the egg, salt and vanilla.

4. In a second bowl whisk together the flours, xantham gum, almond flour and baking soda. Slowly mix the flour mixture into the butter mixture until just combined. Stir in the chocolate chips.

5. Chill the dough in fridge or freezer for at least 10 minutes.

6. Drop spoonfuls of the dough onto the baking sheet. Bake cookies for approx. 10 minutes until just lightly browned on the bottom and still soft (but not liquid-y) on top. Allow to cool for 5 minutes on the sheet and then transfer to a cooling rack.

Notes

Eat in moderation as a treat due to the high sugar and fat content.

Have a nut allergy? The almond flour helps these cookies to stay soft. If necessary you can sub it out with sweet rice flour. However the cookies may be crispier. You could try also baking at a lower temperature (300).

There are two ways to freeze these cookies. You can freeze them after they are baked and cooled. Or you can roll the raw dough into balls, place on a plate and put in the freezer for 20 minutes, and then transfer into a ziploc bag in the freezer. Then when you want fresh cookies bake the frozen dough for 2 minutes longer than the usual time.

Don't have access to lots of gluten-free flours? I have also successfully made these cookies using Bob's Red Mills 1-to-1 Gluten Free flour (which is rice flour not bean flour based) and almond flour. Use 3/4 cup and 2 tablespoons of the gluten-free flour blend in place of the white rice flour, sweet/glutinous rice flour and tapioca starch.

Chicken Fingers

Prep Time: 15 mins

Cook Time: 6 mins

Total Time: 21 mins

Servings: 4 people

Calories: 507 kcal

Ingredients

- 1/2 cup uncooked quinoa (rinsed and dried)
- 1/4 cup freshly grated parmesan
- 1 tsp dried thyme
- salt and pepper to taste
- 1 tsp dried parsley (crumbled)
- 1/4 cup rice flour
- 2 eggs
- 2-3 chicken breasts

- 2 tbsp olive oil

Instructions

1. Place quinoa, parmesan, thyme, salt and pepper, and parsley in a food processor and pulse until it becomes powdery (most of the quinoa should still be intact). Transfer to a plate and set aside.

2. Place eggs in a small bowl and beat them lightly with a fork. Place rice flour on a plate and set both aside.

3. Slice chicken breasts into 1/4-1/2 inch strips (depending on how large you want your chicken fingers). One at a time, dredge your chicken slices through the rice flour, then dip them in the egg to coat them, and finally, through the quinoa mixture. Pat down on the chicken strip to make sure the quinoa is on firmly before removing it from the mix.

4. Once all your chicken strips have been coated, heat up your frying pan and warm 1 tbsp of olive oil. Once the pan is thoroughly heated, add half the chicken strips to the pan. Cook for

6 minutes, turning once. Add the remaining oil as needed.

5. Once the chicken strips have cooked through, transfer them to a wire rack to drain/cool. Continue with the second batch.

Notes

Tiny pieces of quinoa may come off of your chicken strips and burn in the oil. This isn't a problem in the first batch, but they may leave a burnt taste in the oil that will increase the more batches you complete. For this reason, depending on how much space is in my dishwasher, I either wash my pan in between uses or use two frying pans. The added benefit of using two frying pans is that you will finish both batches simultaneously.

One Pan Chicken Dinner Bake

A little butter and Italian herbs make chicken, potatoes, and vegetables tender and delicious.

Prep Time: 10 minutes

Cook Time: 1 hour 15 minutes

Total Time: 1 hour 25 minutes

Servings: 4

Ingredients

- 1 to 1-1/2 lb. boneless, skinless chicken thighs
- 1 lb. potatoes, scrubbed and diced into 1" pieces
- 1 cup frozen green beans
- 1 cup frozen carrots
- 1/4 cup unsalted butter, melted
- 1 teaspoon kosher salt
- 1 teaspoon Italian herb seasoning (I like Frontier)
- 1/2 teaspoon ground black pepper
- 1/4 cup sliced scallions, green parts only

Instructions

1. Preheat oven to 350 degrees F. Spray a 13″ x 9″ baking pan with olive oil cooking spray.

2. Place the chicken thighs down the long middle of the baking pan. Place potatoes on one side of the chicken and green beans and carrots on the other side.

3. Combine the melted butter with the salt, Italian herbs and pepper. Drizzle over the chicken, potatoes and vegetables. Sprinkle with the scallions.

4. Tightly cover pan with aluminum foil and bake for 1 hour to 1 hour and 15 minutes, or until chicken is done and potatoes and veggies are tender. Serve.

Mini Paleo Salmon Cakes & A Lermony Herb Aoili

Prep Time: 15 minutes

Cook Time: 30 minutes

Yield : 10 Servings

Ingredients

- 2 1/4 cups | 12 oz. cooked salmon, flaked
- 1/4 cup mashed or pureed sweet potato or white potatoes, see notes
- 4 green onions, green parts only for low FODMAP, chopped
- 1 tablespoon fresh parsley, chopped
- 1 tablespoon dijon mustard
- 1 teaspoon lemon zest
- 1 tablespoon lemon juice
- 3 tablespoons capers, liquid drained
- 1 egg, beaten
- 3/4 teaspoon sea salt
- 1/2 teaspoon ground black pepper
- Lemon wedges for serving

LEMON HERB AIOLI

- 1 egg yolk
- 1 tablespoon fresh lemon juice
- 1/2 teaspoon dijion mustard
- 1/2 cup garlic infused olive oil for low FODMAP or regular olive oil
- 1 large clove garlic, omit for low FODMAP
- 1 tablespoons fresh parsley, chopped
- 1 teaspoon fresh dill, chopped

Instructions

1. Preheat the oven to 350°/180°C
2. In a large mixing bowl, add all of the salmon cake ingredients. Mix everything together with a fork util combined. Form mini patties, about 3 inches in diameter and place on the baking tray. Bake for 25-30 minutes or until firm and browned on the sides. Make sure to flip the patties over in the oven halfway through cook time.

LEMON HERB AIOLI

1. While the salmon cakes are baking make the aioli. The easiest way to make this is with an immersion blender but you can also make this in a food processor, blender, or using an electric mixer.

2. Place the egg yolk, 1/2 of the lemon juice, and mustard in a small bowl or blender/processor. Start whisking/blending everything together until the mixture thickens. Then gradually pour in the olive oil. It's important to add the oil slowly because adding too much too soon will result in a runny or cuddled aioli. As the mixture thickens, add more oil until you have a thick, creamy mayo.

3. Add the remaining lemon juice along with the garlic, parsley, and dill and mix in by hand. Taste and season with salt if needed. Transfer the aioli to a small bowl and serve with the salmon cakes. Store left overs in an airtight container in the fridge for up to a week.

Notes

Makes 10-12 small patties

If you don't have any mashed potatoes on hand you can make it easily by peeling and chopping 1 large potato (white or sweet) and placing the chopped pieces in a small pan. Cover the potatoes in 1 inch of water and bring to a boil on a high heat. Reduce the temperature and cover. Let heat for 15 minutes of until you can easily pierce the potatoes with a fork. Drain the potatoes and place in bowl. Mash with a fork until no lumps remain.

Nutrition

Amount Per Serving:

- Calories: 61
- Cholesterol: 35mg
- Sodium: 281mg
- Carbohydrates: 1g
- Protein: 7g

Spicy Lemon Pasta With Shrimp

This Spicy Lemon Pasta is made with gluten-free linguini, spinach, and protein-packed shrimp flavored with lemon juice, butter, and a kick of red pepper flakes. It's perfect for an easy weeknight meal or simple stay-at-home date night dinner.

Prep Time: 5 minutes

Cook Time: 25 minutes

Total Time: 30 minutes

Yield: 4

Ingredients

- 1 (8-ounce) box gluten-free linguini (like Ancient Harvest® Supergrain Pasta™ Linguine)
- 1 tablespoon garlic-infused olive oil
- 4 tablespoons butter (or ghee), divided
- 1 to 1 ¼ pound uncooked large shrimp, peeled and deveined
- 1 teaspoon low FODMAP Italian seasoning
- ¼ teaspoon red pepper flakes
- 4 cups spinach

- 2 tablespoons fresh lemon juice
- 2 tablespoon parsley or chives, minced
- Salt and pepper

Instructions

1. Cook the gluten-free pasta according to the package instructions. Drain, toss with a little olive oil to prevent sticking, and set aside.
2. In a large pot, heat the olive oil and 1 tablespoon butter. Add the shrimp and cook until the shrimp start to turn pink; flipping once. Once the shrimp are almost cooked, stir in the Italian seasoning, red pepper flakes, and spinach. Cook, stirring occasionally, until the spinach is wilted.
3. Add the cooked pasta to the shrimp and spinach mixture. Add the remaining 3 tablespoons butter; stir until the butter is melted and everything is well mixed.
4. Top with lemon juice, fresh herbs, salt, and pepper. Serve warm.

Chocolate Orange Chia Pudding

Chocolate Orange Chia Pudding whipped together in a pinch and is perfect for breakfast and dessert alike.

Prep Time: 1 hour 5 minutes

Total Time: 1 hour 5 minutes

Ingredients

- 1 cup dairy free milk of your choice, 240 ml
- ¼ cup chia seeds, 40 grams
- 3 tablespoons cocoa powder
- 1 teaspoon vanilla extract
- 1 tablespoon juice from an orange
- 1 teaspoon orange zest
- 1-2 tablespoon sweetener of your choice, maple syrup, honey, agave etc

Instructions

1. In a jar or container large combine all the ingredients. Whisk until combined.
2. Cover and refrigerate at least an hour or overnight.

3. Top with orange slices, chocolate chips, more zest, or whatever you would like.

Notes

Prep time is about 5 minutes but these need to be left in the fridge at least 3 hours

Use maple syrup for low FODMAP

Nutrition

Yield: 2 SERVINGS

Amount Per Serving:

- Calories: 175
- Saturated Fat: 1g
- Sodium: 168mg
- Carbohydrates: 21g
- Fiber: 10g
- Sugar: 7g
- Protien: 5g

Low FODMAP Nachos

Prep Time: 10 mins

Cook Time:; 10 mins

Total Time: 20 mins

Course: Appetizer, Lunch, Main Course

Servings: 4 servings

Calories: 574 kcal

Ingredients

- 1 bag tortilla chips (gluten-free, unsalted)
- 1/2 lb prepared low FODMAP taco beef
- 1 cup cheddar cheese (lactose-free, shredded)
- 1/2 cup kalamata olives (sliced)
- 1/2 cup lettuce (shredded)
- 1 common tomato (diced)
- 2 green onions (green parts only, diced)
- 1/4 cup sour cream (lactose-free)

Instructions

1. Preheat the oven to 350 degrees and line a baking sheet with aluminum foil. Place a single

layer of chips on your baking sheet and sprinkle with 1/3 cheese and 1/3 taco meat. Make a second layer of chips and sprinkle with 1/3 of cheese, 1/3 taco meat, and 1/3 of olives.

2. Add a final layer of chips and cover with remaining cheese, meat and 1/3 olives. Bake for 5 minutes (or until cheese has melted).

3. Remove nachos from oven and top with lettuce, tomatoes, green onions and remaining 1/3 olives. Place sour cream on the side for the best results. Serve warm.

Thai Coconut Lime Soup

Prep Time: 10 mins

Cook Time: 15 mins

Yield: 5 servings

Ingredients

- 1 Tbsp extra virgin olive oil
- 2 small zucchini, chopped
- 1 red bell pepper, chopped
- 4 carrots, chopped
- 1 potato, washed and chopped
- zest and juice of 1 lime
- 1/4 cup chives, chopped
- 2 tsp ground ginger
- 2 cans lite coconut milk (I prefer Trader Joe's brand)
- 3 Tbsp low sodium Tamari
- 1/4 tsp black pepper
- 4 cups vegetable stock (I used homemade but priced an average box of stock)
- optional, fresh basil for garnish

Instructions

1. Heat the olive oil in a medium pot over medium heat. Add the zucchini, bell pepper, carrots, and potato cooking for 2-3 minutes until they are slightly tender.

2. Add the lime zest, lime juice, chives, ginger, coconut milk, tamari, and broth/stock. Stir and cover, bringing the soup to a boil over high heat. Once the soup is boiling, reduce the heat to low and allow to simmer for 10-15 minutes.

3. To serve: serve as is, garnish with fresh basil or serve over brown jasmine rice or cauliflower rice.

Nutrition

Serving Size: 1/5 of recipe

- Calories: 220
- Sugar: 8 g
- Sodium: 820 mg
- Fat: 11 g
- Carbohydrates: 28 g
- Protein: 3 g

Veggie-Packed Low FODMAP Soup

YIELDS 14

Prep Time: 60 min

Cook Time: 1 hr, 10 min

Ingredients

- 1 Tbs olive oil
- 3 tsp smoked paprika
- 2 tsp cumin
- 1 1/2 tsp chili powder
- 6 medium-large carrots, sliced
- 1/4 c water
- 10 c water
- 15 oz. can salt-free diced tomatoes
- 6 oz. can salt-free tomato paste
- 3 Tbs low sodium soy sauce or tamari
- 3 Tbs lemon juice
- 1 Tbs pure maple syrup
- 1 tsp salt
- black pepper to taste
- 1 c uncooked quinoa

- 6 c collard greens, loosely packed, big stems removed (prep these during cooking)

Instructions

1. Add the oil to a large cooking pot.
2. Add the paprika, cumin and chili powder.
3. Turn the heat up to medium. Add the carrots and the 1/4 c water.
4. Put a lid on the pot and let cook about 10 minutes, stirring occasionally. Stem the greens while the carrots cook.
5. Stir in the rest of the ingredients.
6. Raise the heat to med-high. Lid the pot and bring the soup to a boil (about 8 mins).
7. Turn the heat down to medium, uncover and let simmer about 30-35 minutes.

Skinny Pizza Margherita

We've bumped up the nutrition--and kept all the flavor--of this traditional Italian pizza with tomato, sliced mozzarella, basil, and olive oil.

Prep Time: 5min

Cook Time: 20min

Number of Servings: 8

Ingredients

- 1 recipe Quinoa-Flaxseed Pizza Dough
- 1 recipe Better-than-Pesto Puree
- 1 cup grape tomatoes, halved lengthwise
- 4 ounces soft goat cheese, crumbled

Directions

1. Raise the oven rack to the highest level, then
1. preheat oven to 400° F. If using a pizza stone,
2. place it in the oven to preheat.
2. Place the dough on a pizza screen or preheated
3. stone, spread with the pesto, then scatter the
4. tomatoes and cheese across the top.

3. Bake until the dough is nicely browned and

5. crispy, 18 to 20 minutes.

Note: Pizza pans vary in size. We base our recipes

on a 16-inch pan with eight slices per pie.

Nutrition

Servings Per Recipe: 8

Amount Per Serving

- Calories: 219.9
- Total Fat: 9.7 g
- Cholesterol: 3.3 mg
- Sodium: 181.6 mg
- Total Carbs: 28.0 g
- Dietary Fiber: 2.7 g
- Protein: 5.7 g

Tapenade and Spinach Pasta

Tired of the same old red sauce from a jar? Try this instead.

Prep Time: 12min

Cook Time: 4min

Number of Servings: 4

Ingredients

- 2 t olive oil
- 1/2 cup Tapenade
- 1/2 c Oven Dried Tomatoes
- 2 cups (cooked) whole wheat pasta (cooked with no salt or oil)
- 1/2 cup cooking liquid from the pasta
- 2 cups spinach, larger stems removed
- 2 oz parmesan cheese, shaved

Directions

1. Heat oil in a large saute pan. Once hot, add tapenade and oven roasted tomatoes and saute for 2 minutes.

2. Add spinach and continue to saute for another minute. Add hot pasta and reserved cooking liquid; continue to cook an additional 3 minutes, stirring pan.

Nutrition

Servings Per Recipe: 4

Amount Per Serving

- Calories: 223.1
- Total Fat: 9.3 g
- Cholesterol: 11.2 mg
- Sodium: 276.5 mg
- Total Carbs: 24.1 g
- Dietary Fiber: 1.5 g
- Protein: 10.8 g

Stuffed Chicken Breasts with Olive Tapenade, Tomatoes, and Feta

Make this chicken the next you have company for dinner, and they'll swear you hired caterers. It tastes like it came from a restaurant, but for much less money and effort.

Prep Time: 5min

Cook Time: 15min

Number of Servings: 4

Ingredients

- 1 T canola or olive oil
- 1 pound (16 ounces) chicken breasts (2 breasts cut in half)
- 1/2 c Oven Dried Tomatoes, diced
- 6 T Tapenade
- 4 oz feta cheese

Tips: By using homemade tapenade and roasted tomatoes instead of buying them at the supermarket, you're cutting the cost of this meal in half.

I made this dish with feta, but if you prefer a less salty cheese, use soft goat cheese.

Directions

1. Preheat oven to 350 degrees. Place chicken breast halves between two sheets of wax or parchment paper; pound with a meat mallet or rolling pin to a quarter inch of thickness. Place 1 ounce of cheese, 2 T diced tomatoes, and about 1 1/2 T tapenade on each piece of chicken.
2. Roll up like a jelly roll. Heat the oil over medium-high in a large oven-safe saute pan; once hot, add the meat to sear on all sides. Once the meat is browned on all sides, transfer the entire pan to the preheated oven.
3. Roast for 15 minutes, until meat is cooked and no longer pink inside. Remember to have a hot pad in your hand when you remove the pan from the oven—the handles get hot! Allow meat to rest 3-4 minutes before cutting.
4. Makes 4 servings with 3 ounces of cooked meat.

Nutrition

Servings Per Recipe: 4

Amount Per Serving

- Calories: 269.6
- Total Fat: 14.7 g
- Cholesterol: 95.3 mg
- Sodium: 377.8 mg
- Total Carbs: 2.9 g
- Dietary Fiber: 0.0 g
- Protein: 30.4 g

Perfect Grilled Turkey Sandwich

CookTime: 5min

Number of Servings: 1

Ingredients

- 2 slices whole wheat bread
- 2 oz sliced white meat turkey
- 1 slice reduced-fat Swiss cheese

- 2 leaves green leaf lettuce, torn
- 1 tablespoon Cranberry Relish
- nonstick cooking spray

Directions

1. Preheat a skillet to moderate heat. Spray one side of each piece of bread with nonstick cooking spray. Spread the cranberry relish on the opposite sides of the bread.
2. Place the sprayed side onto the heat. Place the turkey on the pan with the cheese directly on top to warm the meat and cheese; once warm place on top of one of the slices of bread.
3. Place the lettuce on the other slice and sandwich the two slices together. Grill until both sides are golden brown.

Nutrition

Servings Per Recipe: 1

Amount Per Serving

- Calories: 477.5
- Total Fat: 14.9 g

- Cholesterol: 56.7 mg
- Sodium: 479.2 mg
- Total Carbs: 55.3 g
- Dietary Fiber: 5.9 g
- Protein: 32.2 g

Beef and Blue Sandwich

Sandwiches so good, you'll think someone brought home takeout from your neighborhood deli!

PrepareTime: 5min

Number of Servings: 4

Ingredients

- 12 oz (4 servings) Beef Roast, sliced thinly (or another lean beef roast)
- 4 sandwich thins or buns
- 1/4 c plain Greek yogurt
- 2 T blue cheese, crumbled
- 2 c green leaf lettuce
- 1/2 c Caramelized Onions

Tips

Forget grabbing deli sandwiches on the way home from work. You can feed a family of four gourmet, healthy roast beef sandwiches, complete with sweet caramelized onions and creamy bleu cheese dressing, for about $8. That's $2 a sandwich--just try to spend that little at a deli!

Serve with a piece of fruit and a cup of skim milk, and you've got a healthy dinner in no time flat.

You'll still have four servings of roast left. Use them to make Vegetable Beef Soup. These sandwiches can be eaten hot or cold. Try toasting the sandwich thins for added texture.

Serve with a piece of fruit and a cup of skim milk, and you've got a healthy dinner in no time flat.

Directions

1. Prepare the blue cheese sauce by gently combining the blue cheese and Greek yogurt. Layer between the bread the lettuce, beef, onions, and dressing.

Makes 4 sandwiches

Nutrition

Servings Per Recipe: 4

Amount Per Serving

- Calories: 325.0
- Total Fat: 9.8 g
- Cholesterol: 79.6 mg
- Sodium: 358.9 mg
- Total Carbs: 27.7 g
- Dietary Fiber: 5.7 g
- Protein: 33.5 g

Beef Roast with Broccolini and Sweet Potatoes

Prep Time: 30min

Cook Time: 15min

Number of Servings: 4

Ingredients

- 12 oz (4 servings) Beef Roast
- 2 c sweet potatoes, baked or steamed (about 2 large sweet potatoes)
- 2 c broccolini, washed and trimmed (1 bunch)
- 4 t almonds, slivered
- 1/2 lemon, juiced
- 8 T (4 servings) Caramelized Onions
- pinch black pepper

Tips

A quick broccolini side dish and a steamed or baked sweet potato round out the meal. Don't forget a cup of milk!

Broccolini is similar to broccoli, with long thin stems and tender florets. You can substitute asparagus, broccoli or green beans in this recipe.

Directions

1. Microwave or bake the sweet potatoes until tender.

2. Steam or simmer broccolini in water until just tender. immediately place the broccolini in a bowl filled with ice water to stop the cooking. Slice the warmed meat. Heat a non-stick saute pan to medium high heat.

3. Add drained broccolini to the warmed pan. Saute for two minutes. Add almonds and continue to cook for one minute. Remove the pan from heat; add lemon juice and season with pinch of black pepper.

To serve: Place 3 oz meat (about the size of the palm of your hand) on a plate. Top with 2 T caramelized onions. Serve with 1/2 c broccolini and 1/2 c sweet potatoes.

Nutrition

Servings Per Recipe: 4

Amount Per Serving

- Calories: 341.6
- Total Fat: 10.9 g
- Cholesterol: 75.6 mg
- Sodium: 102.5 mg

- Total Carbs: 29.6 g
- Dietary Fiber: 5.8 g
- Protein: 31.1 g

Cheesecake

This is a cheese-cake like dessert. Use any flavored geletin you like. I sprinkles some sugar free cookie crumbs on top.

Minutes to Prepare: 10

Number of Servings: 8

Ingredients

- 1 cup boiling water
- 1 small envelope sugar free flavored geletin (Such as Jell-O)
- 1 6 oz container greek style yogurt (such as Fage) - you can also use plain nonfat yogurt, just strain it first until it's thick and creamy
- 2 8oz packages Low Fat cream cheese
- 2 Tbl Splenda to taste

Directions

1. Mix gelatin with boiling water until disolved. Mix in yogurt and cream cheese until thoroughly mixed together - be patient, it takes a lot of mixing. Add splenda to taste.
2. Let set at least 4 hours or over night. Garnish with fruit, sugar free cookie crumbs or whipped cream. (these are not included in stats).

Nutrition

Servings Per Recipe: 8

Amount Per Serving

- Calories: 155.6
- Total Fat: 10.6 g
- Cholesterol: 33.7 mg
- Sodium: 178.1 mg
- Total Carbs: 5.6 g
- Dietary Fiber: 0.0 g
- Protein: 8.9 g

Lemon Curd

Minutes to Prepare: 5

Minutes to Cook: 15

Number of Servings: 20

Ingredients

- 55g Butter
- 225g Sugar
- 2 Large Eggs - beaten
- Juice and finely grated zest of 2 lemons (or 4 limes)

Tips

When it's cold, store in the fridge - it will last about 1 month.

Directions

1. Put a bowl over a pan of simmering water, and add the butter and sugar until dissolved. Add the lemon/lime juice and zest, and then the eggs whisking as you add them to prevent curdling.

2. Let it cook gently stirring until it is thick and like custard (be patient it takes about 10 - 15 minutes!). Take off the heat and put into a suitable jar.

Nutrition

Servings Per Recipe: 20

Amount Per Serving

- Calories: 72.4
- Total Fat: 2.8 g
- Cholesterol: 24.4 mg
- Sodium: 23.2 mg
- Total Carbs: 12.4 g
- Dietary Fiber: 0.5 g
- Protein: 0.8 g

Veggie Pizza on Whole-Wheat Crust with Feta and Mozzarella Cheeses

A kickin' vegetarian pizza! It's extra good because it's made on a whole-wheat crust!

Minutes to Prepare: 10

Minutes to Cook: 12

Number of Servings: 16

Ingredients

- For one cookie sheet size pizza use:
- 1 (7.5 ounce) can pizza sauce
- 1/2 tbsp. olive oil
- black Pepper to taste
- 1/4 cup onions, chopped
- 1 red bell pepper, chopped
- 6 cloves garlic, chopped
- 2/3 cup sliced mushrooms
- 1 cup spinach, fresh, torn
- 1 large tomato, chopped
- 2/3 cup black olives, sliced
- 1/2 cup feta cheese, crumbled

- 2 cups mozzarella cheese, shredded
- 1 tsp. canola oil

Tips

You can also make this into individual size pizzas.

Directions

1. Pre-heat oven (375F).
2. Using a large skillet or wok (I prefer the wok), saute all the vegetables for a few minutes(except the spinach and tomatoes) in the 1/2 tbsp. of olive oil with a bit of black pepper.
3. Add the tomatoes and spinach, and saute for a minute or two more, or until the spinach wilts and shrinks down a bit. Remove vegetables from the heat.
4. Roll the pizza dough out onto a large, OILED cookie sheet.
5. Spread the can of pizza sauce on the prepared pizza dough.
6. Add a bit of the shredded mozzarella cheese to the prepared crust.

7. Evenly spread the sauteed vegetables over the crust.

8. Spread the black olives over the crust.

9. Crumble the feta cheese evenly over the crust.

10. Top with the remaining mozzarella cheese.

11. Bake in the pre-heated oven for 11 - 13 minutes.

12. Remove from oven, let stand a few minutes, and slice into 16 equal pieces.

13. Enjoy! :)

Nutrition

Servings Per Recipe: 16

Amount Per Serving

- Calories: 171.7
- Total Fat: 7.6 g
- Cholesterol: 12.9 mg
- Sodium: 484.6 mg
- Total Carbs: 19.0 g
- Dietary Fiber: 3.1 g
- Protein: 7.6 g

Beef Bottom Round Roast

Minutes to Prepare: 5

Minutes to Cook: 480

Number of Servings: 6

Ingredients

Beef, bottom round, 2 lb

Directions

Put in Crock Pot on high and cook 8 hrs

Nutrition

Servings Per Recipe: 6

Amount Per Serving

- Calories: 208.7
- Total Fat: 7.1 g
- Cholesterol: 89.2 mg
- Sodium: 190.8 mg
- Total Carbs: 0.7 g
- Dietary Fiber: 0.1 g
- Protein: 33.1 g

Mexican Pizza

This Mexican pizza is a tasty alternative to traditional pizza. Add grilled chicken or cooked shrimp to change this up!

Prep Time: 10

Minutes to Cook: 15

Number of Servings: 12

Ingredients

- 1 c salsa
- 1 14.5 ounce can fat-free refried beans
- 2 T ground cumin
- 1 small onion, sliced
- 1 bell pepper (any color), sliced
- handful fresh cilantro, chopped
- 1 avocado, diced
- 3/4 c low fat sour cream
- 2 c low fat cheddar cheese

NOTE: You can use a regular premade pizza crust to save time! Just adjust the nutrition info!

Directions

1. Preheat oven to 425 degrees Fahrenheit. Bake crusts for about 7 minutes. Remove from oven and spread 1/2 can of beans on each crust, following with half the salsa, cheese, onions, and peppers. Sprinkle on cumin, then place in oven and bake until crust is golden brown and cheese is melted, about 8 minutes.
2. Slice each pizza into six pieces, then top with cilantro, some avocado and 1 T lowfat sour cream. Drizzle on hot sauce (optional)!

Nutrition

Servings Per Recipe: 12

Amount Per Serving

- Calories: 203.9
- Total Fat: 5.7 g
- Cholesterol: 9.9 mg
- Sodium: 423.2 mg
- Total Carbs: 29.0 g
- Dietary Fiber: 3.6 g
- Protein: 11.0 g

Taco Soup

Top this soup with toasted tortilla strips and serve with lime wedges and avocado slices.

Minutes to Prepare: 5

Minutes to Cook: 20

Number of Servings: 6

Ingredients

- 16 ounces extra lean ground beef
- 1 small yellow onion, chopped (about 1/2 cup)
- 1 recipe Taco Seasoning
- 1 (14.5 ounce) can no salt added tomato sauce
- 1 (14.5 ounce) diced tomatoes with green chilies
- 1 (14.5 ounce) dark kidney beans, drained and rinsed
- 1 cup frozen or canned corn kernels
- 1/2 cup chickpeas, drained and rinsed, mashed

Tips

Just before serving, squeeze in the juice of half a lime for a kick.

Directions

1. Brown the ground beef and onion in a large saucepan over medium heat. Blot any excess grease with a paper towel, then add the taco seasoning. Cook for one minute, then add the tomato sauce, diced tomatoes, kidney beans, and one cup water.
2. Reduce heat to medium-low, and simmer for 10 minutes.
3. Add the corn and mashed garbanzo beans, and simmer five more minutes.
4. Serve immediately. Makes six (1 cup) servings.

Nutrition

Amount Per Serving

- Calories: 290.7
- Total Fat: 13.7 g
- Cholesterol: 52.2 mg
- Sodium: 311.3 mg
- Total Carbs: 24.3 g
- Dietary Fiber: 6.5 g
- Protein: 20.6 g

Crispy Faux-Fried Mexican Chicken

I love faux frying foods using panko. This crunchy, spicy chicken would be great on a taco salad.

Minutes to Prepare: 5

Minutes to Cook: 20

Number of Servings: 4

Ingredients

- 1 pound boneless, skinless chicken breasts, pounded until uniform in thickness
- 1 recipe Taco Seasoning
- 1/4 teaspoon salt
- 1 cup panko bread crumbs
- 1 cup low-sodium salsa

Tips If you can't find panko, use crushed baked tortilla chips.

Directions

1. Preheat the oven to 375 degrees.
2. Combine the panko, taco seasoning and salt in a shallow dish.

3. Remove any fat from the chicken breasts. Pull the tenderloin away from the breast; it is on the under side of the breast. Slice the remaining breast into one inch strips. You should get 4 strips from each breast. Spray each strip with nonstick cooking spray, then dip into the bread crumbs to coat the entire surface. Transfer the chicken to a baking sheet. Bake for 20 minutes or until the meat reaches 165 degrees. Serve with salsa.

Nutrition

Servings Per Recipe: 4

Amount Per Serving

- Calories: 221.8
- Total Fat: 3.8 g
- Cholesterol: 70.2 mg
- Sodium: 436.7 mg
- Total Carbs: 19.5 g
- Dietary Fiber: 3.2 g
- Protein: 29.7 g

Meatloaf Cupcakes with Mashed Potato Frosting

Minutes to Prepare: 10

Minutes to Cook: 30

Number of Servings: 12

Ingredients

- Meatloaf Cupcakes
- 2 pounds extra lean (96%) ground beef
- 1 cup panko (Japanese breadcrumbs)
- 2 egg whites
- 1 teaspoon Worcestershire sauce
- 1/2 medium onion, finely chopped (about 1/2 cup)
- 3/4 teaspoon McCormick 25% less sodium steak seasoning
- 3 cups mashed potatoes (We used this recipe.)
- 2 tablespoons chopped flat-leaf parsley
- 1/4 cup reduced-sodium ketchup
- 12 grape tomatoes

Tips

Feel free to skip the parsley and tomato if your kids are picky. You could also top with gravy!

If you don't eat red meat, use ground turkey.

Directions

SERVES 12 ~ 1 meatloaf cupcake per person

1. Preheat the oven to 375 degrees F.
2. Combine all the meatloaf ingredients in a large bowl. Use a half-cup measure to scoop the meat into muffin tins coated with cooking spray.
3. Bake for 20 minutes, or until the meat reaches an internal temperature of 160 degrees F.
4. While the meatloaves are cooking, prepare your mashed potatoes.
5. Transfer the mashed potatoes to a large resealable bag. Snip off one corner of the bag.
6. To serve, place one meatloaf on a plate, then pipe the mashed potatoes (about 1/4 cup) on top.

7. Sprinkle with parsley (optional), drizzle with ketchup, and top each with a grape tomato.

Nutrition

Servings Per Recipe: 12

Amount Per Serving

- Calories: 253.3
- Total Fat: 13.2 g
- Cholesterol: 52.7 mg
- Sodium: 217.4 mg
- Total Carbs: 14.8 g
- Dietary Fiber: 0.8 g
- Protein: 17.6 g

Roasted Beet Salad with Goat Cheese and Walnuts

Prep Time: 30min

Minutes to Cook: 45

Number of Servings: 6

Ingredients

- 1 pound beets, without greens (save greens for the recipe "Beet Greens with Pine Nuts")
- 2 1/2 tablespoons olive oil
- Kosher salt and freshly ground black pepper
- 1/3 cup chopped walnuts
- 4 ounces fresh goat cheese, at room temperature
- 1/4 cup skim milk
- 1 teaspoon chopped fresh chives
- 1/4 cup chopped fresh parsley

Directions

1. Preheat the oven to 425°F.
2. Scrub the beets and place on a large piece of aluminum foil. Toss with 1 tablespoon of the

olive oil and a generous pinch of salt and pepper. Fold the foil to create a packet for the beets and place the packet on a baking sheet. Place in the oven and cook for 45 minutes to 1 hour, until the tip of a paring knife slides easily into the beets. When cool enough to handle, trim, peel, and cut into wedges.

3. While the beets are cooking, place the walnuts on a baking sheet and toast in the oven until fragrant, 8 to 10 minutes. Remove from the oven, let cool for 5 minutes, and roughly chop.

4. In a small bowl, combine the goat cheese, milk, and chives. Stir with a fork to make a thick sauce. Season to taste with salt and pepper.

5. To assemble, spoon the goat cheese sauce on each plate. Top the sauce with beets, toasted walnuts, and parsley. Season the beets with salt and pepper and drizzle with the remaining 11/2 tablespoons of oil.

Nutrition

Servings Per Recipe: 6

Amount Per Serving

- Calories: 183.1
- Total Fat: 14.2 g
- Cholesterol: 8.9 mg
- Sodium: 139.3 mg
- Total Carbs: 9.6 g
- Dietary Fiber: 2.8 g
- Protein: 6.2 g

Seared Scallops with Minted Pea Puree

Not only is this dish pretty on the plate, it's quick and easy to make.

Minutes to Prepare: 5

Minutes to Cook: 5

Number of Servings: 4

Ingredients

- 1 12-ounce bag frozen peas, about 2 cups
- 1 garlic clove, sliced in half
- 1 1/2 cups vegetable stock, no salt added
- 1/3 bunch flat-leaf parsley, leaves only, about 3/4 cup
- 1 tablespoon lemon juice
- 4 mint leaves
- 1/2 teaspoon Lower Sodium Seasoning Blend
- 1/2 pound sea scallops, rinsed and patted dry

Tips

Don't overcrowd the pan or your scallops will simmer rather than sear, which means you won't get that crispy brown exterior. Depending on your pan, you may need to cook in two batches. Why are some scallops so bright and white and others yellow? Purveyors often soak scallops in a solution of sodium tripolyphosphate to brighten their color and extend shelf life. Unfortunately, this can make the scallops rubbery and lose some of their natural nutty flavor. As a consumer, be aware of the difference. You will find both dry scallops not soaked in the solution and wet, which have been brined in the salt solution. If you pick up the brined variety, give them a rinse before cooking.

Directions

1. Place the peas, garlic, and stock in a medium size saucepan over high heat. Bring to a boil and cook for two minutes. Remove from heat and add the parsley, lemon juice and mint. Puree in a blender or using an immersion blender.

2. While peas are cooking, prepare the scallops. Pat the scallops on both sides dry with a paper or lint-free cotton towel. Sprinkle seasoning blend over each scallop. Spray each scallop with a generous layer of nonstick cooking spray.

3. Heat a sauté pan or cast-iron skillet over high heat. When the pan is piping hot, add the scallops. Do not move them once you put them in the pan. Cook for two minutes on each side, spraying the top side with nonstick cooking spray before you flip them.

4. Serve warm. Pour a 1/4 cup of pea puree into a soup plate or dish and top with 3 seared scallops.

5. Serve with couscous or brown rice.

Serving Size: makes 4 servings, 1/4 cup puree with 3 scallops per serving

Nutrition

Servings Per Recipe: 4

Amount Per Serving

- Calories: 172.2
- Total Fat: 1.4 g
- Cholesterol: 35.0 mg
- Sodium: 294.8 mg
- Total Carbs: 16.2 g
- Dietary Fiber: 4.0 g
- Protein: 21.8 g

Chicken Fajita Stuffed Peppers

Minutes to Prepare: 60

Minutes to Cook: 20

Number of Servings: 4

Ingredients

- 1 batch (1 tablespoon) No Salt Fajita Rub
- 1 lime, zested and juiced
- 1 teaspoon vegetable oil
- 16 ounces boneless chicken breasts cut into strips
- 1 large sweet or yellow onion, sliced
- 4 roasted bell peppers or red chili peppers*
- 1/2 cup fresh corn
- 1 cup black beans, rinsed and drained
- 16 grape or cherry tomatoes, sliced
- 2 tablespoon cilantro, chopped
- 1/4 cup chopped cilantro

Tips

Craving crunch? Serve this meal inside raw bell pepper halves! You can also cook this meal on the grill--use a cast-iron grill pan or slice the chicken into strips after it cooks.

Directions

1. Combine the rub, lime zest and juice, and the oil. Pour over the meat, cover and refrigerate for 1 hour or overnight.

2. Place a cast iron or nonstick skillet over medium-high heat. Sauté the onions for 10 minutes, until light golden brown in color, then remove from the pan and set aside. Add chicken to the same pan and saute until cooked through, about 8 minutes. Add the cooked onions, corn, beans, and tomatoes to the pan, stir and cook for one minute. Remove from heat.

3. Place one pepper on a dinner plate, fill with one cup of chicken and vegetables, then top with a heaping tablespoon of the Avocado Cream and cilantro.

Serving Size: Makes 4 servings.

Nutrition

Servings Per Recipe: 4

Amount Per Serving

- Calories: 339.1
- Total Fat: 9.9 g
- Cholesterol: 73.4 mg
- Sodium: 137.8 mg
- Total Carbs: 30.5 g
- Dietary Fiber: 7.4 g
- Protein: 31.8 g

Better Breakfast Casserole

This make-ahead breakfast is perfect for busy mornings or Sunday brunches. And it has half the calories and 1/3 the fat of the original.

Prep Time: 20min

Minutes to Cook: 35

Number of Servings: 8

Ingredients

- 8 ounces (1 recipe) low-sodium breakfast sausage
- 1 bell pepper, chopped (about 1 cup)
- 1 medium onion, chopped (about 1/2 cup)
- 4 ounces mushrooms, sliced (about 1 cup)
- 1 garlic clove, minced
- 1/4 teaspoon red pepper flakes
- 8 eggs
- 3 cups skim milk
- 5 cups whole-grain bakery-style bread, crusts removed and cubed
- 2/3 cup shredded low-fat pepper Jack or Cheddar cheese

Directions

1. Preheat the oven to 350 degrees F if you're making this in the morning rather than the night before.
2. Coat a 9"x13" baking dish with nonstick cooking spray.
3. Cook the sausage in a nonstick skillet over medium heat. Break up the meat into bite-size

chunks as it cooks. When the meat is about halfway cooked, add the pepper and onions. Cook for three minutes, until the vegetables start to soften, then add the mushrooms and garlic. Cook another two minutes, until the mushrooms have started to brown. Add the red pepper flakes and remove from heat.

4. Transfer the veggies and meat to a medium bowl to speed up the cooling process.

5. While the meat and veggies are cooling, combine eggs with milk in a medium mixing bowl.

6. Layer three cups of the bread in the bottom of the baking dish. Spoon the veggies and sausage over the bread, then sprinkle on half the cheese.

7. Carefully pour the eggs and milk into the dish, then top with the remaining bread cubes and cheese.

8. Use the back of a serving spoon to press down on the layers to help the bread soak up the eggs.

9. Cover the dish and refrigerate for up to 24 hours.

10. When you're ready to bake the dish, preheat the oven to 350 degrees.

11. Bake the casserole 35-40 minutes, until the eggs are no longer runny and the bread is golden brown.

Serving Size: Makes 8 servings

Nutrition

Servings Per Recipe: 8

Amount Per Serving

- Calories: 249.3
- Total Fat: 11.8 g
- Cholesterol: 208.6 mg
- Sodium: 247.8 mg
- Total Carbs: 15.4 g
- Dietary Fiber: 2.1 g
- Protein: 19.5 g

Chicken Leftover Tostada

Minutes to Prepare: 5

Minutes to Cook: 5

Number of Servings: 4

Ingredients

- 2 servings (2 cups) Slow Cooker Provencal Chicken and Beans
- 4 8-inch corn tostadas
- 4 c mixed salad greens
- 3/4 c tomato salsa
- 1/2 c monterey jack cheese, shredded

Some grocery stores carry tostadas, which are slightly drier and crispier than tortillas. If you can't find them, use corn tortillas--or your favorite kind of wrap.

Directions

1. Preheat oven to broiler setting. Place tortillas on a sheet pan. Layer on 1/2 cup of the bean mixture then salsa and 1/8 cup (1 ounce) of cheese.

2. Heat under broiler just until the cheese melts. Place a cup of mixed greens on top of each tostada and serve.

Nutrition

Servings Per Recipe: 4

Amount Per Serving

- Calories: 262.7
- Total Fat: 8.6 g
- Cholesterol: 45.6 mg
- Sodium: 865.0 mg
- Total Carbs: 24.6 g
- Dietary Fiber: 5.3 g
- Protein: 21.2 g

Chicken Nachos

Prep Time: 5

Minutes to Cook: 8

Number of Servings: 8

Ingredients

- 2 servings (2 cups) Slow Cooker Provencal Chicken and Beans
- 4 ounces tortilla chips
- 1 1/2 cups tomato salsa
- 1 cup shredded Monterey jack cheese

Tips

Top with shredded lettuce, reduced-fat sour cream, and diced tomatoes and avocado.

Directions

1. Preheat oven to 400 degrees. Layer the chips in an oven proof dish. Top with the meat, beans, salsa and cheese.
2. Bake until cheese is the bubbly, about 8-10 minutes.

Nutrition

Servings Per Recipe: 8

Amount Per Serving

- Calories: 189.5
- Total Fat: 8.8 g
- Cholesterol: 29.1 mg
- Sodium: 557.8 mg
- Total Carbs: 15.6 g
- Dietary Fiber: 3.5 g
- Protein: 12.6 g

Faux Fried Cheese Sticks

Minutes to Prepare: 3

Minutes to Cook: 10

Number of Servings: 4

Ingredients

- 4 reduced-fat string cheese sticks

- 1 tablespoon flour
- 1 cup panko (Japanese bread crumbs)
- 1/2 cup egg substitute (or 2 egg whites)
- 1 1/2 tablespoon Italian Herb Seasoning Blend

Directions

1. Preheat the oven to 375 degrees. Spray a baking sheet with cooking spray. Pour the flour onto a small plate.
2. Cut the cheese sticks in half. Roll the cheese sticks in the flour.
3. Place the breadcrumbs and Italian herbs in a small container with a lid or zip-top bag and set aside.
4. Pour the egg substitute into a shallow dish. Using one hand, roll the floured cheese sticks in the egg mixture. One at a time, using your other (dry) hand, transfer the cheese sticks to the bread crumb mixture and shake to coat. Using the dry hand, remove from the crumb mixture and place on the baking pan.
5. Continue until all the cheese sticks are breaded.

6. Spritz each cheese stick with cooking spray. Bake for 10 minutes or until cheese is bubbly and melted.

7. If desired, dunk these cheese sticks in low-sodium tomato sauce (calories not included).

Makes 4 two-stick servings.

Nutrition

Servings Per Recipe: 4

Amount Per Serving

- Calories: 145.2
- Total Fat: 2.8 g
- Cholesterol: 10.0 mg
- Sodium: 340.2 mg
- Total Carbs: 15.1 g
- Dietary Fiber: 0.6 g
- Protein: 15.4 g

Mini Sweet Potato Tarts

Minutes to Prepare: 5

Minutes to Cook: 20

Number of Servings: 12

Ingredients

- 8 oz phyllo dough, thawed
- 2 c sweet potato, steamed or roasted, flesh only
- 1/2 c dark brown sugar
- 1/2 t salt
- 1/2 t pumpkin pie spice mix, plus additional 1/2 t for dusting
- 1/4 c low-fat evaporated milk
- 1 t vanilla
- 1/2 c egg substitute or 2 egg whites
- 1/2 c fat free whipped topping

Tips

To boost the fiber, you can look for whole-wheat phyllo dough, which is available in the healthy food freezer section of many grocery stores.

Directions

1. Preheat oven to 350 degrees. Spray 24 mini muffin cups with nonstick cooking spray. Remove phyllo dough from packaging. Slice into 1 inch strips, then cut each strip into 2 inch segments. Using 3 layers at a time, fill the cups, spraying cooking spray between each layer. Repeat process three times. Remove skin from sweet potatoes and allow to cool to room temperature. Place sweet potatoes, sugar, spice mix, milk, and vanilla in the bowl of a food processor. Blend until smooth. Add eggs and blend just to incorporate. Fill cups to the top of the muffin pan.
2. Bake 18-20 minutes, until custard is set and pastry starts to brown. Once cooled, top with 1 teaspoon of fat-free whipped topping and a dusting of pumpkin pie spice mix.

Makes 12 servings (two tarts per serving).

Nutrition

Servings Per Recipe: 12

Amount Per Serving

- Calories: 151.0
- Total Fat: 2.0 g
- Cholesterol: 1.7 mg
- Sodium: 221.8 mg
- Total Carbs: 33.0 g
- Dietary Fiber: 1.7 g
- Protein: 3.3 g

Vegetable Beef Soup

Minutes to Prepare: 10

Minutes to Cook: 25

Number of Servings: 8

Ingredients

1. 3 carrots, peeled and chopped

2. 1 onion, chopped

3. 4 stalks celery, chopped

4. 1 (14.5-ounce can) no salt added diced tomatoes

5. 4 cups low-sodium beef stock

6. 12 ounces cooked beef sirloin, cubed into 1/2 to 3/4 inch cubes (or 4 servings of Beef Roast)

7. 1/2 teaspoon black pepper

8. 1 tablespoon Thai chili sauce (optional, or to taste)

9. Directions

10. Coat a large, heavy saucepan with nonstick cooking spray. Set over medium heat.

11. When the pan is hot, add the carrots and onions. Cook for about 2 minutes. Add the celery to the pan; continue another 3 minutes.

12. Add the tomatoes and the stock. Turn the heat to high, bring to a boil and then reduce heat to low.

13. Simmer the soup for 15 minutes. Add the beef, pepper, and Thai hot sauce, and cook for three minutes.

14. Remove from heat and serve immediately.

Makes 8 one cup servings.

Nutrition

Servings Per Recipe: 8

Amount Per Serving

- Calories: 119.6
- Total Fat: 3.6 g
- Cholesterol: 37.8 mg
- Sodium: 379.0 mg
- Total Carbs: 4.7 g
- Dietary Fiber: 0.9 g
- Protein: 15.9 g

Oven-Roasted Tomatoes

Load up on Roma tomatoes when they're in season, then dry them in the oven to intensify their flavor and savor them all year round.

Prep Time: 5

Minutes to Cook: 90

Number of Servings: 12

Ingredients

- 3 pounds plum (Roma) tomatoes
- 2 tablespoons extra virgin olive oil
- 3 cloves garlic, minced
- 1 t basil, dried
- 2 t Italian Seasoning
- 1/2 t black pepper, cracked

Tips

Make large batches when tomatoes are in season, then freeze them for use during winter. Serve them in a sauce over whole wheat pasta, on a sandwich or in a green salad.

They're quite versatile and affordable. The entire recipe costs about $4, which means each serving is about 32 cents. If you use tomatoes from your own garden, this recipe is even cheaper.

Directions

1. Preheat oven to 275 degrees. Remove the top and bottom of the tomatoes. Slice to remove the seed area.
2. Discard the inner flesh and seeds. Cut the slices into 2 inch strips. Combine all remaining ingredients and toss with the tomatoes. Roast for 2 hours on a roasting rack. Remove from oven and allow to cool.

1/4 cup per serving.

Nutrition

Servings Per Recipe: 12

Amount Per Serving

- Calories: 28.9
- Total Fat: 2.4 g
- Cholesterol: 0.0 mg

- Sodium: 3.4 mg

- Total Carbs: 2.0 g

- Dietary Fiber: 0.4 g

- Protein: 0.4 g

Mint Chocolate Chip-Oat Cookies

You'll never know these cookies are lower in fat! Customize your cookies by using any flavor of "chips" you prefer!

Minutes to Prepare: 20

Minutes to Cook: 10

Number of Servings: 40

Ingredients

- 4 Tbsp "I Can't Believe It's Not Butter Cooking and Baking Blend"

- 1/3 cup low fat cream cheese (1/3 less fat)

- 1 cup light brown sugar, packed

- 2 large egg yolks
- 3/4 tsp vanilla extract
- 1/2 cup oat flour
- 1/2 cup all purpose flour
- 1/3 cup whole wheat flour
- 3/4 tsp baking soda
- 1/4 tsp salt
- 5 ounces dark chocolate and mint chips

NOTE: To make oat flour, place oats in a food processor or blender until they achieve a flourlike consistency.

Directions

1. Preheat oven to 350 degrees Fahrenheit.
2. Prepare baking pans by spraying with canola oil spray. You may also line pans with parchment paper or use a silicone baking liner.
3. Cream the "butter," cream cheese and brown sugar on high speed using a mixer. Once the mixture is fluffy, reduce the speed to low and add the egg yolks and vanilla. Mix until combined. Combine the the flours, baking soda, salt, and chips in a bowl. Add to the

butter mixture and mix by hand until well blended.

4. Drop heaping teaspoons onto a baking sheet about 2 inches apart. Flatten lightly with the bottom of a glass that has been moistened with water.

5. Bake 6-7 minutes. Rotate the pans and bake until lightly browned, about another 3 minutes. Be careful not to overbake. Cool and store in tightly sealed container.

Nutrition

Servings Per Recipe: 40

Amount Per Serving

- Calories: 69.2
- Total Fat: 2.9 g
- Cholesterol: 11.4 mg
- Sodium: 53.6 mg
- Total Carbs: 12.5 g
- Dietary Fiber: 0.3 g
- Protein: 0.8 g

Slow Cooker Salsa Chicken

Minutes to Prepare: 5

Minutes to Cook: 480

Number of Servings: 8

Ingredients

- 2 pounds (32 ounces) chicken breasts, boneless and skinless
- 1 cup salsa, homemade or purchased
- 1 cup petite diced canned tomatoes (choose low-sodium)
- 2 tablespoons Taco Seasoning
- 1 cup onions, diced fine
- 1/2 cup celery diced fine
- 1/2 cup carrots, shredded
- 3 tablespoons sour cream, reduced fat

Directions

1. Salsa Chicken is easy to make; just put all the ingredients in a slow cooker and let the machine do the work. There are infinite

variations, and your family is guaranteed to like each one.

2. 6-8 hours to prepare; 15 minutes of active cooking time

3. Makes 8 one-cup servings of chicken

4. Place the chicken in a slow cooker. Sprinkle the taco seasoning over the meat then layer the vegetables and salsa on top. Pour a half cup water over the mixture, set on low and cook for 6-8 hours. The meat is cooked when it shreds or reaches an internal temperature of 165°F. When ready to serve, break up the chicken with two forks then stir in the sour cream.

Makes eight 1 cup servings

Nutrition

Servings Per Recipe: 8

Amount Per Serving

- Calories: 177.5
- Total Fat: 4.1 g
- Cholesterol: 72.4 mg

- Sodium: 240.3 mg
- Total Carbs: 7.3 g
- Dietary Fiber: 2.1 g
- Protein: 27.2 g

Chicken-Veggie Quesadillas with Ranch Yogurt Sauce

Prep Time:10

Minutes to Cook: 10

Number of Servings: 4

Ingredients

- 1/4 cup low-fat plain Greek yogurt
- 2 tsp Ranch Seasoning Blend
- 12 ounces boneless and skinless chicken breast
- 1 tsp canola oil
- 2 red or orange bell peppers, top and bottom removed, cored and seeded
- 4 whole-wheat tortillas

- 2 tomatoes, diced
- 1/2 cup shredded Monterey or pepper Jack cheese

Directions

1. In a small bowl, make the sauce by combining the yogurt and 1/2 teaspoon of the seasoning blend. Cover and chill in the refrigerator.
2. Place the chicken into a plastic bag. Using a meat mallet or rolling pin, pound out the meat to 1/4-inch thickness. Add oil and remaining seasoning blend to the bag. Marinate meat 10 minutes or up to 8 hours.
3. Place a cast-iron skillet or nonstick skillet over moderate heat. Once warmed, add the peppers. Sear the peppers by pressing down on them, 2 to 3 minutes. Remove from heat, let cool slightly, and dice.
4. Place the chicken in the skillet (discard the marinade), and cook over moderate-high heat for 4 to 5 minutes. Turn, and continue to cook until internal temperature reaches 165° F, about 5 minutes more. Remove the meat from

the skillet, let cool slightly, and dice. Wipe out the skillet with paper towels.

5. Reheat the skillet to moderate heat. Build the quesadillas one at a time by placing a tortilla in the pan, then layering on half of the chicken, peppers, tomatoes, and cheese. Top with a second tortilla and cook for 2 minutes on each side until the cheese melts. Remove the cooked quesadilla to a cutting board. To serve, cut each quesadilla in half, with a pizza wheel if you have one. Serve with the ranch sauce.

Nutrition

Servings Per Recipe: 4

Amount Per Serving

- Calories: 242.5
- Total Fat: 9.1 g
- Cholesterol: 66.2 mg
- Sodium: 227.6 mg
- Total Carbs: 14.6 g
- Dietary Fiber: 1.8 g
- Protein: 25.6 g